"Today is the first day of the
rest of your life "

INDEX

DISCLAIMER

The methods I am about to share with you that were responsible for a full recovery from my PND are intended to tell the story of my recovery, and the steps I would recommend to beat PND from my personal experience only. This ebook is not medical advice.

I am not a doctor, and recommend that you seek qualified medical advice regarding your PND treatment.

I recovered from PND without the use of any medication however I am in no way suggesting whether you should or should not take anti-depressants as I am not medically qualified to give you that advice.

A Special Note For You

Congratulations on taking the first steps to recovery. It isn't any wonder that women can have low moods, as having a baby is such a life changing event.

It takes enormous strength, courage and self sacrifice to give birth and raise children in the world today. Please remember to give yourself credit for this every day.

The first thing I want to say to you which is imperative to your recovery is this:

"DO NOT BE AFRAID OF POST NATAL DEPRESSION"

Post Natal Depression will not last, and it is my intention to help you recover quickly. Trust that what you are going through is an illness that is treatable and that you will return to normality.
The next thing I want to stress to you is this:

"PUT ALL STRATEGIES INTO PRACTICE"

Actively try to make changes in your life. Reading the following methods alone may not get the

results you want. Make a commitment to put every method into practice, whether in your current state of mind you believe it will help or not.

And finally:

" START THE IMMEDIATE ACTIONS IN SECTION 6 - TODAY! "

You must start now! Do not delay, as you will start to see results.

I hope with all my heart that my information can help you in a big way, and wish you a full and fast recovery. Remember I am just an email away, so please write to me and let me know how you are going.

I am hoping to expand my help into a forum in the future so that we can all give support to each other.

My Story

I had no signs of PND with my first child 10 years ago. It wasn't until I had my second child and I was 38 yrs old that I experienced severe post natal depression. It started with baby blues , crying in the first week after birth of my daughter Amy, and never really went away. I had lots of problems with breast feeding, in the first 3 weeks, had mastitis which required daily laser treatment at the hospital and I literally did not have more than 1-2 hrs sleep at a time. I was extremely tired and felt very down which I assumed would be perfectly normal considering the circumstances.

I then put Amy on formula which solved a lot of problems and started getting at least 4-5 hrs sleep at a time which was much better. The low feelings however persisted. I came to a decision when Amy was 6 weeks old that I needed to return to full time work. I felt very upset and angry that I had given up a career and could not cope with a life of changing nappies and making bottles. I felt devastated and was in tears often. Returning to work was all I wanted to do. I didn't care that I wouldn't be with my newborn baby all day, I desperately wanted to escape the depressive feelings and find some peace.

I returned to full time work and spent 3 months running around like a crazy woman. My mornings started at 5am getting ready to take Amy to my mothers and go to work. I returned home with Amy between 6.30 - 7.oo pm. By the time we had finished dinner and dishes, ironed clothes for the next day, made lunches for myself, husband and 10yr old daughter for the following day it was 10'oclock at night. I would collapse, go to bed (still get up in the night for Amy waking up) and do it all again the next day. I eventually had a break down after 3 months and could not continue. I went to my local doctor in tears telling him that I had taken on too much. It was at this point that he diagnosed me with PND.

I couldn't believe it. Infact, I didn't really believe him. I was confident that I had only taken on too much to handle and rejected his suggestion of anti-depressants.

I was then at home again all day with my baby, while my husband went to work and my eldest daughter to school. I started to feel scared of being alone but didn't know why. I felt anxious when my husband was leaving as though I doubted my ability to cope at home alone. What was I scared of? I had no idea. It didn't make sense. Then over days & weeks I progressively and secretly felt worse and worse. I felt trapped in my own home, I couldn't keep up with the housework, I felt hatred for myself, I didn't know how to manage my time in the day . I didn't want to go out, I didn't want to take phone calls, I didn't return emails. I felt like a useless wife and useless mother and useless friend.

I got to the stage where every time I went out I was filled with such anxiety and panic, I felt separated from everyone and everything like I was walking around in a foreign land. People would talk to me and I would answer them, but it felt like it wasn't really me, it was someone else. I had disappeared, or been taken over by some weird existence. I desperately wanted to escape these feelings but didn't know how.

Each day I would wake up and wished that I hadn't. Each morning I dreaded the day ahead. I could no longer get in touch with any feelings of happiness or joy. I was numb. There was no such thing as happiness anymore, I wondered how I ever felt joy in the past and cried believing that I had lost it forever.

Each day I crawled out of bed because I had to. My family were depending on me and this was my only purpose for existence.

I soon started to question whether maybe my family could infact get on with life without me. I was useless to them anyway I thought, and even more so now a burden as I wasn't coping. My husband was under more pressure trying to comfort me and keep the family stable and all I seemed to do was yell and scream at everyone for the smallest of things. What good was I?
I looked into my beautiful Amy's eyes and secretly thought that she would be too young to remember me or be upset if I was no longer around.

My husband would be upset , but would cope because he was strong.

My eldest 10yr old daughter however, I did not think would cope with the loss of me. Due to circumstances, I had been the only one thing in her life to this point that was consistent and I knew how much she depended on me and how much she would be devastated and probably ruined for the rest of her life if I were gone. I realised I could never leave.

I never actually got to the point of deciding that suicide was an answer, but I can tell you that I was heading that way. I contemplated what life would be like for everyone I knew if I were gone. Somewhere at this point, co-incidentally my husband had taken steps to force me into looking for help.

I wanted the help. I wanted to feel better, I wanted to feel normal again. I desperately wanted to feel the slightest bit of joy. I enrolled in a 9 week group program that wasn't starting for another 6 months. I honestly didn't know how I was going to cope for another 6 months on my own. At this point I went back to a doctor I hadn't seen for a while. He was my family doctor of many years that I trusted immensely. I had stopped seeing him as we had moved out of the area and was more than half an hours' drive away. This doctor strongly encouraged me to commence anti-depressants. This doctor had advised me in the past to throw cough medicine in the bin and was against any drugs that were not necessary, so I considered what he was suggesting. I tried an anti-depressant one morning and had a reaction to the medication. I felt confused and delusionary for a couple of hours. This experience made my decision that I was not going to take anti-depressants at all.

Through all of this dilemma, I had forgotten about all the self help books that I had read over the previous 10 years. I have always had a strong interest in self development and the power of the mind . When I came to this realisation, I became empowered to tackle this PND head on, armed with strategies that I put together from all that I had learnt.

From that point I have never looked back. Day by day I improved. On my own I managed to beat the fear of PND and wipe out the symptoms. My 9 week course was also an invaluable contribution, and the self-discovery journey was amazing.

During my recovery period I decided to do a web design course which has given me the skills to be able to share my information with the world.
It is my hope that I can reach and help many others that are in a similar position to what I was.

It is my hope that I can reach both women who are already receiving treatment as well as women who are reluctant to seek treatment outside their own front doorstep.

It is my hope that I can give some support to those women who no doubt are feeling isolated and alone, because you are not alone, there are millions of women around the world going through the same thing, experiencing the same feelings. The more you realise how common it is, and connect with others who feel the same, the easier it will be to understand and overcome PND without fear.

It is my hope that the following information will take you through your own journey to recovery. I have condensed all the successful strategies that I put into place from my own self help study, and some strategies learnt in my 9 week PND program.

Best Wishes,
Your Friend and Mentor
Shona

Introduction
An Understanding of PND

What is Post Natal Depression?

Adjusting to a significant life changing event such as having a baby can be difficult and commonly cause depression. Not only do women have to cope with a major life change, they also have to cope with the additional day to day stress of a new baby. Some women may experience depression during pregnancy which is referred to as 'antenatal depression'. Postnatal depression is more common and is experienced in the months after giving birth.

PND vs BABY BLUES vs POSTNATAL PSYCHOSIS

It is important to recognize the difference between Postnatal Depression, Baby Blues and Postnatal Psychosis.

The 'baby blues' occur between 3-10 days after giving birth, are common and affect 80% of women. Symptoms include tearfulness, and a feeling of overwhelmness. The baby blues usually disappears within a few days.

Postnatal Depression may develop between 1 – 12 months after the birth of a baby. Approx 16% of women are affected in Australia. Symptoms which will be detailed on the next page can develop suddenly or gradually.

Postnatal Psychosis is rarer, affecting 1 in 500 women after childbirth. Symtoms may be present in the first week or so after giving birth and may include thought disturbances, hallucinations, paranoia and delusions. Postnatal Psychosis is an emergency and medical help should be sought immediately.

What are the symptoms of PND?

Behavioural changes that last for more than 2 weeks may be an indication of depression:

- Moodiness that is out of character

- Increased irritability

- Finding it hard to take minor personal criticisms

- Withdrawal from friends and family

- Loss of interest in food, sex, exercise or other pleasurable exercise

- Sleeplessness

- Increased drug/alcohol use

- Staying home from work or school

- Increased physical health complaints (ie fatigue/pain)

- Recklessness

- Slowing down of thoughts and actions

Recovery Overview- Healthy Mind Healthy Body

I have always had a personal interest in self development, and by that I mean developing a positive approach to life and wellbeing.

I have studied many books on positive thinking and mind power and have come to my own conclusions that the quality of our health is dependant on the quality of our thoughts.

"Healthy Mind , Healthy Body" is my motto.

You will notice that there is a huge emphasis these days on looking after our bodies. Health problems are emerging out of control all over the globe, things such as obesity and diabetes to mention a few. Medical associations everywhere are recommending that we exercise regularly. Schools are playing a more important role these days to ensure that children are also exercising on a regular basis.

But there is something missing here in my opinion. Where is anyone here suggesting that we also exercise our minds?
Is mental health not part of total health? If we go to the gym to exercise our bodies for an hour a day, our bodies will be fit and strong, but our minds may still be weak. We may still be prone to negative thinking, and the way we react and cope with life events is based on how we think, and what we say to ourselves.

This concept may be new to you.

Lets talk about the power of the mind with Post Natal Depression. Postnatal Depression is a 'mood disorder'.

Our moods and feelings are created by our 'thoughts'.

For example: IF you allow yourself to think about and dwell on a very hurtful experience from the past, you will notice that you will start to have feelings of sadness. The good news is, that you have a choice about whether

you want to think about it or not, can choose to think of something happier thus can avoid feelings of sadness.

In my opinion depression comes about by a build up of negative thoughts. Many of these thoughts have become subconscious thoughts as during our development as a child we develop patterns of thinking. We may not even realise what our inner voice is saying to ourselves, putting ourselves down, always thinking the worst etc etc. The spiral of negative thinking becomes so bad that the result is a mood disorder-depression.

You can lift yourself out of this by re-programming the mind to think positive thoughts. At first a lot of time and commitment is required to think in a positive way, until it becomes automatic and then the ability to feel happiness and joy will return.

My Steps 1- 10

The following steps are what I followed to re-program my mind and lift the post natal depression. I would recommend following these steps with conviction. At first you will not feel any joy from doing these activities, and this is normal while your mind is going through change, so please persist no matter how much you do not believe in these steps.

Immediate Actions

1. **SEEK PROFESSIONAL HELP**

    If you have not already spoken to your doctor or PND specialist, then I want you to pick up the phone and make an appointment right now. Drop all feelings of embarrassment or not wanting help. In particular I would recommend trying to find a PND group session program where you can connect to others in the same situation. I had no idea that the benefits of doing something like this would help me as much as it did. I felt anxious and embarrassed on the first day, but ended up with such support and wonderful friends.

2. <u>**WRITE YOUR RECOVERY STATEMENT**</u>

This is an extremely powerful exercise and must not be skipped. It is one of the key elements in permanently changing your thought patterns.

1. **I want you to think of three words that describe your worst symptoms of PND. For example 'anxious' , 'afraid', 'sad', 'tired' ,'useless' , 'unorganised' etc .**

2. **Now I want you to write 3 words that describe the opposite to what you have just**

written. These words must describe how you wish you felt. For example 'calm', 'energetic' , 'strong' , 'happy' etc.

3. Now you must put your 3 words from step 2 into the blanks below to create your recovery statement.

   I AM _____, _____ AND _____!

   You may feel silly writing this statement as you do not yet believe what it says. It is the exact opposite of what you feel now. This is done for a reason, so just trust it. The statement I used was "I am happy, healthy and calm"

4. **Write this statement boldly on cardboard or paper and place it in different visible areas around your house.** (this is

optional but must be placed at least in one place in the home ie. Your bedroom, where you will see it every day).

5. **You now must repeat this statement over and over to yourself whenever you have the chance.** You must try your hardest to visualise and feel yourself in this state whilst saying the statement. **Say it out loud and in particular in front of a mirror whenever possible for even greater effectiveness.**

    (you will notice your inner voice(thoughts) trying to tell you that the sentence is not true, and that you are not infact anything like the sentence you are saying. This is very normal and part of the process. You are to ignore this inner voice and talk over it by

repeating the sentence again and again)

6. This exercise will need commitment. You will need to commit to this recovery statement until you notice that the most severe feelings of depression have disappeared. You should notice the low moods become less severe initially (within 7 days), and then lesser and lesser each week, particularly if you combine with step 3.

STEP3: EXERCISE / RECOVERY STATEMENT COMBO

Many studies have been done over the years that indicate that regular exercise is effective in helping to reduce depression. I for one can confirm this to be true in my situation. What I also found to be even more so effective is to combine exercise with my recovery statement.

1. **Check with your doctor what exercise is recommended for yourself and if allowable do one of the following.**
2. **Start walking for at least 30 – 60 mins per day. Get out there with the baby in the pram and keep on walking for as long as you can.**
3. **Whist you are walking, repeat your recovery statement over and over. Do not let any negative thoughts (the inner voice) enter your head. Walk and Talk the recovery statement only!**
4. **If the weather is not good, find another way to exercise. If you enjoy the gym, get on the treadmill, bike or crosstrainer, work**

up a sweat and repeat/
think the recovery
statement with conviction
and determination!

5. Find a way to exercise that
    suits you, find a babysitter
    or crèche if needed, and get
    that recovery statement
    happening whilst you are
    exercising and your
    adrenalin is pumping.

STEP 4: DAILY MOOD CHART

This exercise is going to help you to analyse
your moods and detect any patterns/trends
that trigger a low mood. If you can identify a
cause of a low mood it is much easier to
know what areas of your life to focus on

making a possible change.

1. Make up a chart or table similar to this example that will cover a period of a whole month, starting today.

Week 1		AM	AFTERNOON	PM
DAY 1	Rating			
Comments /Triggers				
DAY 2	Rating			
Comments/Triggers				

1. You are going to rate the morning, afternoon, and evening of every single day of the week with a number between 1 -10.

1= lowest mood

10= high/excellent mood.

2.   Underneath each rating you are going to write down the main event/ reason for the rating.

Here is an example of one of my days

Week 1		AM	AFTERNOON	PM
DAY 1	Rating	3	5	7
Comments /Triggers		Chaotic morning. Husband was running late	Baby slept for an hour. Average afternoon with no events.	Went to my web design course.

As you can see, my lowest point of the day was the morning with a rating of 3. This was triggered by everyone running late in my household which caused me to feel stressed. The afternoon was neither good nor bad. The evening was much better with a rating of 7 as I was able to take a break from the home and go out and attend a course in something that I found interesting. It was also good for me socially as it I was interacting with people and meeting new friends.

This is an excellent activity to complete over the period of a month.

3. **Analyse your triggers for both low and high ratings. Try to include more of the events that are triggering a high mood if possible throughout your week on a regular basis. If you have no high ratings, I want you to focus on the ratings that are higher than the lowest, and do more in this area.**

4. **You will find that over the period of a month you will gain a better understanding of what is going on with your moods and**

hopefully be able to determine the reasons behind some of your low moods.

5. Make a note of events that are triggering your low moods and look for ways that you can make changes in these areas to make it easier. Depending on the issue you may be able to ask your partner, a friend or relative for assistance, or seek counselling. If you are attending a PND group program your facilitator may offer suggestions to help you in this area.

Step 5: 14 x 14

This is an exercise that we are going to do over a period of 14 days. The purpose of this exercise is to wipe out a negative belief that you may have about yourself.

1. Ask yourself this question. "What is it about myself that I hate the most or that is causing me the most stress ? "

You will more than likely have more than one answer. We are going to concentrate on one issue at a time. You may have issues for example such as ' I cannot cope being a mother', 'I am unorganised', 'I can't bond with my baby', ' I am fat', what ever it is, write it down.

2. Focus on one issue only, eg. 'I am fat' and write down some powerful words that describe exactly how you would like to be. Eg 'attractive', 'sexy', 'slim', 'toned'. Or "organised, calm, relaxed, happy, social "etc etc

3. Pretend that you have already achieved all of these things that you wrote down in step 2, and write a sentence starting with "I AM" or " I EASILY" that states that this is exactly how you are now. (even though it is not yet true)

Examples of some sentences may be:

"I AM a sexy, slim mum with beautiful toned legs"
"I EASILY cope with being a mum"
"I AM always organised"
"I EASILY bond with my baby every minute of the day"
"I AM happy with what I achieve everyday"

4. **Find 30 mins a day where you cannot be disturbed. Get a sheet of paper and down the page write the numbers 1 – 14. Leave a space underneath each numbered point to write a comment.**

5. **Write your sentence down on line number 1. When you are writing the sentence you must write it with belief! This is critical.**
    You should now have a negative

thought about this sentence from your inner voice ie: no your not, this is not true, what a load of rubbish, you've always been fat, what a joke, this is stupid, this wont work etc etc etc.

In the space provided under line 1, quickly write down what the thought was, do not think about it or analyse it, just write it down and move on to line number 2 and repeat (write your sentence again with belief!)

6. **Repeat this process until you have completed your sentence 14 times.**

What this exercise is doing, is re-programming your mind and changing your thought pattern on this issue. By writing down the negative response, you are actually releasing it! You will find that over the process of 14 days there will be less and less negative responses, you may not even get any (in this case just keep going with the positive statements as usual).

7. **Do not make the mistake of thinking that this exercise is silly. It works! Give it time and you will see!**

8. **You can repeat this exercise every 14 days with a new sentence, targeting another negative thought that you would like to change about yourself.**

Step 6: Get Social

Being social is more than likely the last thing you feel like doing. If you felt like I did, you may feel like hiding away from the world right now. However, a small step in the social direction is required for your recovery.

1. **Pick up the phone and organise a social get together for one day this week. This can be as little as meeting someone for a coffee for half an hour. Another option may be to enrol in a mothers group that meets once per week.**

2. **Make sure that the social get together is <u>outside of your home</u>. If you have no transport then get someone to come to you, but <u>go out</u> for a walk.**

3. **Do this at least once per week, every week**!

You may not feel like going, but you must persist in dragging yourself there no matter what. It will help to lift your mood over time, if not immediately.

Step 7: Sunshine & Relaxation

1. Get out into the sunshine at every opportunity. Studies have shown that sunshine actually helps to reduce depression. Try to get at least 15 mins per day if possible. Make sure you <u>do not </u>wear your sunglasses for at least 15 mins.

2. Get hold of some relaxation music and/or classical music cd's. Play them in the background at home, and in the car. This can be used to assist in reducing stress and anxiety.

3. Learn meditation and breathing techniques. This may be available on a book or cd from your local library.

Step 8: Pleasant Activities

A contributing factor to PND can be that we are so busy with family and chores and what ever else may be taking up our time, we barely leave a minute of time to ourselves to focus on something we enjoy or something that gives us a rest.

At this point in time you may have forgotten what it is that you even enjoy anymore, I know I did. It is now time to make some time in each day for yourself.

1. **Plan a minimum of 4 pleasant activites per day for yourself. Plan them the day before preferably.**

2. **What is a pleasant activity? Anything that gives you time out from responsibility.**

    Pleasant activites may be sitting down and having a cup of tea in silence for 15 mins whilst your baby is asleep. Maybe you may ring a friend and have a chat for 10 mins. Maybe your partner can give you time out for half an hour and you can sit and read a magazine or book, or have a relaxing bath. It is crucial that you get even the smallest amount of rest, and time out from chores/housework and other responsibilities.

3. **Let go of any guilt that is accompanied with making time for yourself!**

The housework is a never ending chore, trust me, even if you work non stop all day long, new mess will still be there tomorrow..! Let go of any unfinished responsibility, whether it be home duties or work responsibilities. Being a mother is the hardest job in the world and you deserve a break. Take it for your healths' sake.

Step 9: Thought Switching

Do the preparation for this exercise and use the technique every time you feel yourself getting stressed, angry, anxious , sad, or experiencing any other negative feelings/thoughts towards yourself that makes you feel bad.

1. **Write a list of as many positive things about yourself that you can think of. This list will include both physical aspects and personality traits. Dig very deep to find even the smallest, trivial things about yourself that you like, have achieved or think others may admire**.

Here are some examples:
I like the colour of my eyes
I have nice shiny hair
I am good at listening to other people

My skin is very smooth and nice to touch
I am a good, honest person
People always enjoy my company
I have a nice smile
My teeth are beautifully white
I am excellent at saving money
I am a fantastic cook
I like the way my hair curls naturally
I am a very kind person
I am great at sharing and giving to others

Write down anything and everything that you can think of that is good about **you**. Write at least 31 things, to cover every day of at least 1 month.

2. **Every morning, choose one thing off this list.**
   This is going to be your 'thought switcher' for the day.

3. At any time during the day when you start to get stressed or angry at yourself, <mark>IMMEDIATELY STOP THAT THOUGHT and replace it with your 'thought switcher of the day'</mark>. Say it out loud if appropriate, go to the mirror and say it if possible. Repeat and focus on this positive thought until you notice that it has made an improvement in your mood.

Step 10: Be Determined

1. Do not give up !!

Recovering from post natal depression will not happen instantly but is a process that can happen quicker with commitment and a fighting determination. You may feel as though you are going through a mind battle, and in fact you are, you are changing your negative thought patterns.

When you go to a gym with a personal trainer, you work out your physical body and experience pain and discomfort. In some ways this is similar. It is a work out of the mind and may not always feel comfortable. As with a physical body workout, a mind workout will start to see results too over time. How much time will depend on how much training you put in and how committed you are. There may be times when you feel that the battle of mind is quite difficult, but please persist and have faith that you are winning.

2. You will win !!

I found that by following these steps with vigilance and a strong determination to beat this mood disorder, my severe symptoms initially became less intense. I then noticed that I no longer felt such low moods anymore, but joy in my life was not present either. I'll never forget that first day when I walked into the supermarket to do my weekly food shopping, and all of a sudden I felt the most intense joy. For no apparent reason I was smiling from ear to ear. No I wasn't on drugs! I felt like dancing down the isles, I felt ridiculously overwhelmed with happiness. I knew then that I was a winner.

CONCLUSION

The powers of the mind are still being discovered and debated. It is my strong belief that the power of your mind has the potential to cure depression.

Something important to note is that recovery from depression does not happen in a steady straight line. What I mean by that is it is perfectly normal to have a few great days and then experience a bad day again. The bad days will become less and less overall. I myself experienced a few great weeks in a row, and then had one bad day. Initially I panicked and thought I was going backwards, but infact I was still going forwards. I don't have any bad days anymore.

I hope that the information I have provided gives you great success in bringing happiness and joy back into your life. I would love to hear from anyone who would like to share their story with me, provide feedback or ask for assistance.

Very importantly don't forget to give yourself credit for the wonderful children you are bringing into the world and the self sacrifice you are currently making.

Please make sure that you also encorporate the help of a professional counsellor and/or PND group program to speed up your recovery even further.

My thoughts and best wishes are with you.
Your friend & mentor
Shona